Plant-Based Menu Planner
for Busy Families

A simple quick-start guide to help real people
enjoy healthy and delicious food.

By Christin Bummer
Edited by Dr. Michael Bummer

Table of Contents

About the Author---------------------------------- i

Introduction-- vi

Mother Knows Best: Eat your veggies -----------1

Getting Started: Tips for Jumping Right In ----- 10

Making it Last: Practice Makes Permanent --- 16

Meal Plan for One Week----------------------- 25

Grocery List for One Week -------------------- 42

Another Helping Please! More resources for

follow-up------------------------------------- 50

About the Author

Christin **Bummer** has been sharing her knowledge about a plant-based lifestyle since she adopted it in 2010. Originally known for her popular blog, Beans Not Bambi, she teaches busy people in the real world how to produce delicious food and how to make healthful choices in real life situations.

After being confused and frustrated by rising blood pressure and stubborn extra weight in her late twenties, despite following a low-carb high protein diet as was recommended by so many experts, she eventually found optimal health through a plant-based diet. In a matter of weeks, she brought her cholesterol, blood pressure, and blood glucose into optimal ranges and easily maintained her ideal body weight as a side effect. After a healthy pregnancy she found it difficult to make the same health-promoting food decisions and in 2014 she joined Chef AJ and John Pierre's Ultimate Weight Loss program. Following the principles of calorie density and their management program for processed food addiction, she lost 25 pounds and maintained the weight loss easily.

The excellent nutrition generated energy and a new zest for athletic pursuits. She completed many miles of training runs, two half marathons, and gained a new appreciation for strength training. She fell in love with obstacle course racing and has since completed a Tough Mudder Half, Spartan Sprint, Bone Frog, and two Terrain Races. In 2017 she began The Nourishing Life to reach a broader audience of folks wishing for support with a transition toward a healthier life. What began as a few coaching clients has grown into a supportive community sharing advice and guidance in a private Facebook group. Her passion for sharing information about plant-based health and wellness comes from a genuine desire to bring the same joy and vibrancy to those in her life, including you!

Dr. Michael Bummer is a board-certified OB/GYN who counsels hundreds of patients a month, feeling honored to play a supporting role in one of life's greatest miracles, pregnancy and the birth of a baby. He entered the field of obstetrics and gynecology to help usher new life into this world. Also, gynecology is one of the very few specialties that provides continuity of care through every phase of a woman's life.

He adopted a plant-based lifestyle along with his wife in 2010 and was thrilled to have the chance to counsel his own wife while she was pregnant with their daughter. Despite his passion for and wealth of knowledge on the topic, he doesn't have enough time to educate every single patient about plant-based nutrition. So far he has written prescriptions for patients to follow up with some of his favorite resources such as the Forks Over Knives documentary, the Starch Solution by Dr. John McDougall, and Unprocessed by Chef AJ. He has guided enough patients toward optimal health to see the benefits first-hand, and wanted to share this information with as many people as possible by way of this book.

Introduction

As more and more people are becoming aware of the numerous benefits of a plant-based diet, many people are realizing that food has the ability to help you rediscover your waistline, improve your energy levels, help you sleep better at night, and if done right – you can say goodbye to cravings forever! Every day, more people are adjusting their priorities and completely re-thinking the way that they eat. But... they don't even know where to start. People who were raised to believe that a complete meal consists of a protein, a starch, and a vegetable may feel really lost at first. I get it. I've been there! It seems like you're skipping all the main entrees and living the rest of your life off of the side item menu, right?

Many people accustomed to dining out a lot may be transitioning to a lot more home-cooked meals as they begin to realize that restaurant meals and prepared food just aren't as healthy as we all wish they were. After all, unless it comes out of your own kitchen, there's no way to control exactly what you're eating. Let's face it, keeping a fresh supply of interesting meals on the table can be daunting. Unfortunately, it's enough to stop many well-intended individuals before they even get started. But not you, you're different! You are going to make sure you succeed this time and we are going to help you.

When you're done with this quick-start guide, you will understand precisely what to grab at the grocery store in order to prepare several simple meals that everyone will enjoy. I will show you how to tweak the dishes in a few different ways so that your family may not even realize they're leftovers! I will offer some tried and true recipes and winning food combinations while giving you the template to be more creative on your own if you wish to be. You will understand how to jump right in and more importantly, how to make it last. I hope you never have to pick up another diet book again! I am going to help you incorporate simple tools so you can enjoy the vibrant health you crave without spending all of your time in the kitchen!

Chapter 1:
Mother Knows Best: Eat your veggies

You've heard it a million times, to the point where you probably don't even hear it anymore: Eat Your Veggies! Whether it's your grandmother, your parents, Dr. Oz, your family doctor, or all of the plant-based doctors out there, they're all saying the same thing. And then there are the multitude of diets out there including low carb/high protein like Atkins, paleo, and keto; the Mediterranean diet, the South Beach diet, or high carb, low-fat vegan and whole food plant-based diets, there is only one point they all agree upon: Vegetables are good for you, and you can eat as many as you want.

Every single one of the diets out there, whether long-term lifestyle plans or short-term diets to slim down, all agree on this point. That tells me that it's worth noting and paying attention. Even with consensus established decades ago, the average American's intake of vegetables is dangerously low, and our rates of chronic and acute disease are alarmingly high. According to the Centers for Disease Control and Prevention, "Seven of the top 10 leading causes of death in the United States are due to chronic diseases, and treating people with chronic diseases accounts for 86% of our nation's health care costs." More than one-third of Americans are obese. Not just overweight, obese! Obesity rates have doubled in adults since 1980 and tripled in children. Despite the era of information where we know more than we ever have before, we are sicker than any other time in history.

Why is this?

- *It's too difficult!*
- *I don't like veggies!*
- *I'll stick to the pizza and potato chips, thanks.*
- *I'd rather try the donut diet!*

Pizza, burgers, and chips "taste better" because they're very specifically designed that way. They contain the holy trinity of tasteful bliss: sugar, fat, and salt, in such perfection, and we are wired biologically to prefer these foods. The richer foods found in nature would be higher in calories, so our brains evolved to seek rich, calorie dense food to ensure our survival. Unfortunately, in the modern era, rich food is more than abundant and our brains are ill-equipped for this environment.

This biological predisposition for rich foods has been noted by the food industry and they're using it to their advantage with incredible success. There are scientists in laboratories across the country who have experimented with ingredients to find the "bliss point" in the brain, the point at which you just have to have more. The result is that the famous marketing claim, "Bet ya can't have just one" is as sure as death and taxes. And unless we figure out how to navigate the hot water we're in, death and disability may come much sooner than we'd like to think!

Animal-based food products are well known to be high in fat, high in cholesterol, and completely lacking in micronutrients and fiber. Yes, they contain a lot of protein, but animal-based protein comes at a very high cost to your health. The World Health Organization has classified processed meats (including ham, bacon, sausage, hot dogs, deli meat, etc) as carcinogenic which means they are known to cause cancer. Red meat (beef, pork, lamb, goat, etc) is classified as a "probable carcinogen" which means it might be wise to avoid it until they can decide for sure. Despite successful marketing attempts steering

4

Americans to choose white meat for health benefits, chicken has been shown to have virtually the same amount of cholesterol and saturated fat as beef. I'm not going to get into the ethical considerations here, but suffice it to say that every time you choose produce over animal products, you're checking a box to vote for morality, kindness, and compassion not only for your body but for the earth and for the animals we share it with.

Plant-based foods, on the other hand, are nature's true powerhouse of nutrients. They come in a rainbow of colors, flavors, and textures, and their nutrient profile is just as diverse. A stroll through any produce section in the United States will show you a display of hundreds of options for fresh vegetables. You can even find more in cans and in the freezer section. The colors are representative of their profile of phytonutrients, and the more variety in your diet, the better. You've heard the phrase, "Eat the rainbow" and it refers not to tiny rainbow-colored fruit flavored candies, but to actual fruits and vegetables.

Here are just a few examples:
Red: red bell peppers, red beets, tomatoes, strawberries, watermelon, raspberries, cherries
Orange and yellow: carrots, orange bell peppers, sweet potatoes, bananas, lemon, pumpkin
Greens: spinach, bok choy, kale, collards, romaine, avocado, broccoli, kiwi, celery, zucchini
Blue/Violet: Blueberries, purple grapes, eggplant, purple onions, purple cabbage, blackberries

Each color vegetable and fruit represents a specific set of phytochemicals that have specific benefits. Reds tend to be high in lycopene and anthocyanins which play an important role in heart health and reducing inflammation. Oranges and yellows are high in beta-carotene, potassium, and vitamins A and

C, and are helpful in reducing inflammation and aiding sore muscles in recovery after exercise. Purple foods are high in antioxidants and flavonoids which have been proven to fight certain cancers as well as to deter ulcers and urinary tract infections. Greens are high in magnesium, iron, and calcium and have been proven to prevent and treat cancers such as colon, breast, and bladder. They're also known for improving bone strength and supporting your endothelium which helps protect your entire vascular system to prevent and reverse heart disease. So next time you turn your nose up at a plate of fresh greens... well, shame on you!!

So which color should you eat for breakfast? Which vegetable is the highest in vitamin X? Do you have to eat them in any particular order? Not at all! Despite the confusing headlines and single nutrient claims of media and marketing, you don't need to have an advanced degree to eat healthfully. Quite frankly, many a well-intended healthy eater has gone back to junk food because they got bogged down in the specific details. Don't let that be you! All you need to know is that eating a good variety of vegetables and fresh fruits every day will ensure you have optimal nutrition from a wide variety of sources. You do not need to worry about "food combining" individual nutrients in each meal as we once thought you did. The human body is a remarkable machine. Feed it the right fuel and it can take care of the rest. Your body can store most nutrients and use them as building blocks as needed.

But alas, eating vegetables alone is not enough! You won't get enough calories that way, and you won't feel full. If you've ever tried to go vegan by living on baby carrots and celery sticks, you already know that doesn't last! Trust me, I know folks who have tried. We'll talk more in chapter three about how to make it sustainable and how to make it simply delicious.

Chapter 2:
Getting Started: Tips for Jumping Right In

As Chef AJ has been saying for years, the reason we don't prefer vegetables is simply that we're not eating them enough. We learn to prefer that which we habitually eat. So in order to start liking vegetables, you've got to start eating vegetables and other whole natural plant foods a whole lot more often! I have designed a one-week meal plan to walk you through a sample week to do just that. But first, let's look at some steps for making the transition a little smoother for you.

The very best plan is to have a plan... If you just "try to eat better" you're highly unlikely to succeed. I have to admit that the culture is stacked against you. If you're going to finally remove that stubborn excess weight or free yourself from a life of medications or chronic disease it's going to take a lot more than a half-hearted effort. You're going to be swimming upstream, so to speak, and it certainly does not happen by accident. So give yourself the gift of time to plan. Sit down and plan what you're going to eat, set the recipes out, make a grocery list so you have the corresponding ingredients on hand, and it will give you a much greater chance of success.

Focus on abundance, not lack. This is possibly the biggest stumbling point I hear people struggling with. If you focus on the things you can't have, you're in for an uphill battle. You're going to see a long list of things you used to eat that even though you know they won't serve you, you'll want them anyway. They will cloud your perspective on your new and improved menu. The reality is that there are at least 50 different vegetables commonly available at every grocery store in the US. There are around 15 different kinds of beans, dozens of potatoes

11

and squash varieties each, and a dozen different kinds of grains all commonly available. Abundance is not going to be your problem. Perspective is! Focus on all of the incredible variety of plant foods, consider experimenting with some you never buy at the grocery store, and you'll look at this as an exciting adventure, not a dreadful task.

Start with what you know. I am providing a sample week of plant-based meals and I'll show you how you can eat for a week with just a few recipes. But if you already have some favorite veggies, beans, or full recipes, of course, you should work those in too. Start with what is familiar and branch out from there.

Avoid the recipe rabbit hole. In the beginning, you will have to try new recipes I'm sure. It's ok to look, but don't let yourself fall into the trap of thinking you need 365 new recipes before you start incorporating some into your routine! It's daunting and sure to stop you in your tracks.

You don't have to survive on quinoa (pronounced KEEN-wah) and collard greens with dozens of spices in each recipe in order to be healthy. I'll share some of my favorite resources for recipes. Pick just one or two resources to start and give yourself permission to be boring and repetitive with it for a while! Most people, regardless of their dietary choices, make the same favorite recipes over and over again with only occasional variety. Eating a vegan or whole foods plant-based diet is no different. Just pick a few favorites and get started.

Plan your week and buy the groceries to match. I've heard so many people say that they throw out more spoiled vegetables than they eat fresh ones. This is usually due to the fact that they went grocery shopping or to the farmer's market without a plan, or even worse - hungry! That's a recipe for disaster. If you just buy what's on sale or what looks good to you at the time, there's a strong chance you won't end up using it, especially if you're grabbing new foods you're not used to using. Have you ever picked up a bunch of kale because you heard it's good for you, and then you went home having no idea what to do with it and a week later you threw it out? I have! Planning in advance not only saves you from a lot of food waste but it saves you the mental exercise of having to figure out what to do with it after the fact.

Chapter 3:
Making it Last: Practice
Makes Permanent

Almost everyone embarking on a new style of eating has some level of apprehension about the change. They worry it won't taste good. They worry they won't be able to stick to it. They worry they might get judged for trying and failing - and conclude that it's safer not to even try. But "easier" is all relative, right? Sure it might be more comfortable to stick to your old routines, but how will you feel if you join the ranks of the obese or diabetic? Will that be easy to accept? Is it easy to have to ask for help tying your own shoes because you can no longer bend down and reach them? Is it easy to rely on help taking care of your children because you just suffered a cardiac event and need to take it easy?

Some say they don't have time to eat healthier. Sure it may take more time to cook than to order takeout, but if you choose to have other people prepare your food most of the time, you'll be spending a lot more time visiting doctors and specialists. I'll also be happy to teach some techniques to make food prep faster and more streamlined. Some say it's too expensive to buy healthy food. What's cheaper - mowing your own lawn or hiring a lawn service? Again, if you're ordering a lot of your food from restaurants or eating a lot of processed foods, you are paying someone to prepare it for you. The cost of medications and medical care usually runs inversely to the cost of your groceries. So the more you spend on fresh, healthy food, the less you'll spend on medications down the road.

Be prepared for withdrawal. This is going to be a big transition if you're used to the standard American diet (ironically abbreviated as SAD). By focusing on filling up on fresh produce,

17

you're going to be shifting your diet to foods that are lower in calories. This is a great thing for weight loss and overall health of course but it's also a big switch for your palate. Remember that your brain is hardwired to drive you toward higher calorie foods. Moving away from high-calorie animal foods and processed foods in favor of lower-calorie plant foods is probably going to feel unnatural at first. You're likely to experience cravings and even some withdrawal symptoms in the first few weeks.

The very best way to cope is to be prepared. Expect that you may feel a little worse before you get better. Please trust the process and know that you really are acting in your own best interest. Think about someone trying to quit smoking. In the first few days without a drag, do they feel better right away? No! They feel horrible! They may be tempted to think "geez, my body just seems to do better on cigarettes, I guess I'd better keep smoking them. It just works for me." I've heard it said so many times about meat and dairy - "It just works for me." It might feel like it does in the short term, but sadly I don't think any of us are immune to the internal dangers that animal products pose to our health. The sooner you get through withdrawal, the sooner you will feel better.

Eat enough starch. This is huge and I can't stress it enough. Remember back to the wannabe vegan who tried to live off baby carrots and celery sticks? Even if you could consume them all day every day without going absolutely bonkers from boredom, you could never consume enough to get in a normal calorie load. Let's say you ate a giant plate piled with steamed vegetables for breakfast, lunch, and dinner. And for snacks, you had an apple and a banana twice a day. You might feel pretty full and you'd surely be chewing all throughout the day, so it's not that you're *really* starving yourself. After all, you hardly have time to rest before the next snack comes. However, that would add up to only about 750 to 800 calories. You might be able to do that for a couple days or more, but you will not be able to sustain it, nor should you try to! You will eventually elicit a starvation state where your body clings on to its fat reserves for fear of an ongoing lack of nutrition. So when you finally can't take it anymore, you have a stressful day, and you find yourself standing in front of a checkout counter wallpapered with candy, or driving near your old favorite fast food joint... well, forget about your plans. They're out the window before you can say, "Yes, I sure would like fries with that!" And now that your body is in a starvation state, you can bet it's going to cling to those calories and build up your fat stores in a hurry in case you try to pull another fast one come Monday morning. Can you see where this cycle comes from?

Redefine Normal. Let's face it: If you are making a serious effort trying to be healthy, you are no longer normal. If you are going to succeed in making your dreams a reality, you will somehow have to come to terms with that. You might get funny looks when you make certain requests at a restaurant. You may have friends who stop inviting you out to events because you're making them reflect on their own choices and it makes them uncomfortable. It's really ok, I promise. In a society where it's normal to know someone battling cancer, or someone who suffered a heart attack in their 40's or 50's... I'll take a pass on normal, thank you very much. Now is a good time to evaluate what's more important - standing out as an oddball for eating differently or being the only grandma at the playground who's able to chase her grandkids around - and actually catch them!?

Remember why you started. There's a great anonymous quote that has come across my path on many occasions, usually when I need it most. "When you feel like quitting, think about why you started." I can't stress enough, whether you decide to dip a toe in the water or cannonball into a whole food plant-based lifestyle overnight, you are bound to face obstacles. Planning ahead will help you tremendously. Knowing why you're doing it is absolutely essential. Even the best planning falls by the wayside if you forget why you're even doing all of this.

"Being healthier" is not an end goal in and of itself. So what is your end goal? When you dig deeper, most people say they'd like to be healthier so they can do one of the following:

- Be around longer for their children and grandchildren
- Lose weight to feel better about themselves
- Spend more quality time with their friends and family
- Avoid the disability and disease they've seen loved ones endure
- Remain independent as a senior

Be sure to take the time to think about this. Knowing your "why" will not only help you get started with greater conviction, but it will keep you going when you face challenges.

Chapter 4: Meal Plan for One Week

O K, it's time to dig in! I'm going to show you how to use just 3 breakfast ideas, 2 lunches, and 4 dinner entrée recipes to make enough food to last all week, and how to change it up to keep it interesting. Of course, if you're cooking for 1 person or a family of 6, you'll have to modify the quantities to suit your needs, but you'll get the idea.

Breakfast #1
The Breakfast Bowl

If you're used to cereal or pop tarts and pastries for breakfast, this is my go-to recommendation. It's quick and easy, and very similar to what you're already doing, so it's an easy transition to make. Simply assemble the following ingredients into a bowl and top with your favorite non-dairy milk and a sprinkle of cinnamon.

Ingredients you'll need:

Rolled oats (instant would work here if that's all you have or if rolled oats are too chewy raw)

Raisins

Dried apricots

Chopped walnuts

Non-Dairy Milk (I love Almond - Original or Unsweetened)

Granola or other cereal with as low sugar content as you can find.

Cinnamon

**Bonus points for fresh blueberries, raspberries, blackberries, and ground flaxseed.

The granola or other cereal is just added as a condiment to give some extra flavor and crunch. Perhaps you can start with half oats, half cereal, and wean yourself gradually to less and less cereal. The idea is to limit sources of processed foods and added sugars. Shy away from dried fruits with added sugar (like cranberries, blueberries, mango, etc.) You can find plenty of options without the added sugar, and there's enough natural sugar in the dried fruit. I find the dried fruit is a nice addition here especially for those who are in transition, but fresh berries are even better, and a good target to strive for eventually. The cinnamon is a really nice way to cut back on sugar without noticing it as much.

Breakfast #2
Overnight Oatmeal

There are hundreds of recipes online for overnight oats, and I'll link to a couple of my favorites at the bottom, but the idea is that you can take rolled oats (old fashioned, not instant), and soak them in non-dairy milk, add mashed banana or applesauce, add simple spices, refrigerate overnight, and you've got delicious hearty oats ready and waiting in the morning. And they'll keep easily for a few days. They soak up the milk overnight giving it a nice texture without taking the time to cook. Store individual servings in mason jars and you've got the fastest healthiest grab and go breakfast!

Ingredients you'll need:
Rolled oats

Non-dairy milk of choice - almond, coconut, oat, hemp, or cashew are all good choices. There are often at least 3 versions of each - original, vanilla, and unsweetened. If you haven't yet found a plant-based milk you enjoy, keep trying! There are an enormous variety of choices!

Applesauce or ripe bananas

Cinnamon

Chia seeds or ground flax seeds

Other spices like cardamom, nutmeg, and ginger are nice additions too.

Basic overnight oats recipe for 3-4 servings:

Banana Nut Overnight Oats

1 cup Rolled oats

1 Banana, mashed

1 cup Non-dairy milk

1 Tbsp Chia seeds or ground flax seeds (optional)

1 tsp Cinnamon

½ tsp Cardamom

2 Tbsp Walnuts, chopped

Add all ingredients except walnuts to a mixing bowl, combine. Store in refrigerator overnight. Stir and add chopped walnuts when serving. Serve warm or cold.

If oats aren't your thing, you can try this option with leftover rice or quinoa to mix it up.
For a new twist, try Carrot Cake Overnight Oats from Sharon Palmer, the Plant-based Dietitian.

Breakfast #3
Guilt-Free Homemade Waffles

This was one of my first recipes when I published Beans Not Bambi and it remains one of my most popular. You'll need a waffle iron for this one but if you don't have one, I've provided a couple great pancake recipes as an alternative. These are best fresh and hot but can be made in advance to become a grab 'n go if you're short on time in the mornings and don't want to wait for the weekend to enjoy this treat! Your friends and family will be blown away that these are whole food, healthy "just as tasty" alternatives to a powdered, processed waffle mix!

Ingredients:

2 Tbsp Ground flax seed

6 Tbsp Warm water

2 Ripe bananas

1/4 cup oat milk (soy and almond work great too)

2 1/2 -3 cups Rolled oats

1 tsp Cinnamon

1/2 tsp Vanilla bean powder

1 Tbsp Chia seeds and hemp seeds (optional, to increase protein content)

1 1/2 cup Fresh fruit, chopped. Raspberries, mango, strawberries, and blueberries make for a delightful treat but most fruit will work great.

Combine flaxseed and water in a small bowl, set aside. Mash bananas, add oat milk and continue mashing until smooth. Stir in oats and spices. Stir in flax mixture. Cook in waffle iron as per directions. Top with fresh fruit and serve. Makes 4 classic square waffles.

If you don't have a waffle iron or prefer pancakes anyway, try these recipes from The Big Man's World:

Fluffy Flourless Banana Smoothie Pancakes

Fluffy Low Carb Cinnamon Roll Pancakes

Lunch Recipe #1
Chopped Salad

I know you may not think you need a recipe for salad, but let me tell you - chopping a salad is a game changer! And having the right ingredients will improve it more than you realize. I post a lot of my meals on Instagram and the chopped salads always get the most comments. They're just so darn pretty! Let me share what I have learned. This is NOT your typical garden salad.

1) Start with a wide variety of veggies - carrots, celery, bell peppers, red onion, green onions, broccoli, etc. Add fruit - cherry tomatoes, grapes, berries, apples, etc

2) Add greens - mixed greens, kale, romaine, spinach

3) Chop well - this is the fun part. Great time to get your frustrations out! Here's the knife I use: Wusthof mezzaluna

4) Add starch - chickpeas and brown rice are my favorites, but sweet corn, peas, and a

variety of beans will really change it up nicely and offer some great satiety.

Timesaving TIP: You can pre-chop the initial veggies in a large quantity once a week and store them together in the fridge. Keep the greens and fruit separate and it will all keep well.

Lunch Recipe #2
Buddha Bowl

A Buddha Bowl is a really fun way to combine foods together that you might not otherwise think of as a complete meal. I like to pick a grain (rice, quinoa, oat groats), pick a couple different kinds of vegetables, and some plant protein (think chickpeas, black beans, edamame, or tofu). Pile it all artfully and add a dollop of hummus or some flavored balsamic vinegar. Dig in. You can get as fancy or as plain as you want to, but this makes for a fabulous way to use up some ingredients you may have from last night's dinner, or some staples you always have in the pantry. Here's a sample:

Ingredients:

1 cup Brown rice

2 cups Sautéed zucchini, yellow squash, and cherry tomatoes

½ cup Black beans

2 Tbsp Hummus or avocado

A generous drizzle of coconut balsamic vinegar

Dinner Recipe #1
Instant Pot BBQ Lentils

This recipe was contributed by Johanna Burris Lackey using a BBQ Sauce recipe created by Mairead Reddy, both members of Chef AJ and John Pierre's Ultimate Weight Loss Program.
More on the wonderful Instant Pot here!

This recipe is so simple and easy to make, but what I love as much as the flavor is the fact that it's so versatile. You can eat it straight out of the pot like a chili, over a bed of greens, spooned over a baked potato or baked sweet potato, or you can serve it over toasted buns just like ol' fashioned sloppy joes. This is where planning ahead is key. This makes a large batch that could easily fill the table for 2 dinners and 2 lunches and they could all be different variations on a theme!

Ingredients:

Lentils:

1 pound Dry brown lentils, sorted & rinsed

1 large onion, diced

15-oz can No-salt-added diced tomatoes, drained

Fresh spinach leaves, torn into small pieces, as desired

BBQ Sauce:

6-oz Tomato paste

1 tsp Onion powder

1/4 tsp Allspice, optional if desired

1 tsp Liquid smoke

3-oz Napa Valley Grand Reserve Vinegar

1-oz Lemon juice

Place all ingredients in a medium-sized bowl. Stir with a fork or whisk vigorously until smooth.

Instructions:

Place lentils in Instant Pot and add water to 6 cup mark. Add diced onion. Cook in Instant Pot using

Bean/Chili function and set the timer to 18 minutes. Allow natural pressure release. Make BBQ Sauce while lentils are cooking.

Drain lentils/onions when pressure is released. Place lentils/onions back in Instant Pot to keep warm. Add tomatoes, spinach, and BBQ Sauce. Stir until well mixed.

Serving suggestions:

Dinners:

Over roasted potato, sweet potato, or Japanese sweet potato. Each will add a unique flavor.

Over toasted buns, as you would sloppy joe's topped with ketchup and mustard if desired

Lunches:

Cold in lettuce wraps with fresh chopped tomatoes
Warm or cold plain or topped with avocado slices

Dinner Recipe #2:
Veggie Stir Fry

Ingredients:

Brown rice

Choose 4-5 of your favorite veggies. Options are endless, but these are some of my staples:

Asparagus

Broccoli

Zucchini

Bok choy

Red bell peppers

Onion

Mushrooms

3 Tbsp Soy sauce

2 Tbsp Lemon juice

½" Fresh ginger

1 Clove of garlic

Rice:

Go ahead and get your brown rice cooking first. That way you'll be ready to eat as soon as the veggies are done. You can do boil-in-bag on the stovetop, use an electric rice cooker, or in the Instant Pot I like to do 4 cups brown rice with 5 cups water, manual setting for 12 minutes.

Veggies:

Put everything but the mushrooms in a frying pan or wok on medium-high heat with 2-3 tablespoons of vegetable broth. Any non-oil liquid works here – vinegar, water, red or white wine, soy sauce. "Water-sauté" the veggies for 3 minutes to start the cooking process without making them mushy. Stir frequently and continue adding small amounts of liquid at a time to prevent sticking. Add the mushrooms and sauté for another 2-3 minutes. Just for fun, also add water chestnuts, bamboo shoots, and/or baby corn if you have it.

Sauce:
Add straight to the pan: 2 Tbsp lemon juice (fresh is best), 1 clove of garlic, pressed or minced, and 1/2 inch minced ginger root. Simmer over low heat 3-5 more minutes until the veggies are done to your liking. If you haven't transitioned away from salt yet, you may wish to add soy sauce when serving.

Serve over brown rice for dinner and use the leftovers for the next day's lunch. You can also add the veggies to the top of a garden salad or even have them for breakfast. Save the extra rice for a rice version of morning oatmeal.

Dinner Recipe #3
The Potato Platter

This Potato Platter lunch or dinner is a technique I learned from Chef AJ's Ultimate Weight Loss Program. It's sinfully easy, infinitely variable, and never gets old! It's an easy go-to when having guests or bringing food to someone's house. It's essentially a make-your-own-potato bar and you can put a different theme to the toppings every time or pick a favorite and repeat. The beauty is in the simplicity but you can make it as fancy as you want with the toppings.

Simply bake 1 potato per person (Prick with a fork and bake at 350 degrees for around 60 minutes, until fork tender.) and make a couple extra in case anyone wants seconds (they always do!). While the potatoes are baking, chop up the ingredients and set out in individual bowls so each person can make their own potato. Here are 3 different ideas to get you started, but use your imagination and share

38

your own ideas in the comments too. These can be lunches or dinners. Plan ahead and bake a whole tray of potatoes so you have them for several days.

Burrito / Potato (It's like To-MAY-to / To-MAH-to, get it?)

Black and/or pinto beans

Corn

Salsa or fresh pico de gallo

Sautéed fajita veggies – peppers, mushrooms, onions

Your favorite hot sauce

Veggie Lovers Pizza Potato

Marinara sauce

Sautéed bell peppers, red onions, and mushrooms

Steamed broccoli, zucchini, or any other veggie you love

Black olives

Pineapple

Mediterranean Tater

Hummus

Kalamata olives

Chopped spinach (wilted or fresh)

Cherry tomatoes, chopped

Cucumbers, chopped

Green onions, chopped

Sample menu for one week:

	Mon	Tue	Wed	Thu	Fri	Sat	Sun
Bfast	Breakfast Bowl	Banana Nut Overnight Oats	Breakfast Bowl	Banana Nut Overnight Oats	Breakfast Bowl	Guilt-Free Waffles	Cinnamon Roll Pancakes
Lunch	Chopped Salad	BBQ Lentils in lettuce wraps	Chopped Salad	Buddha Bowl	Chopped Salad	Buddha Bowl	Chopped Salad
Dinner	BBQ Lentils over sweet potato fries	Veggie Stir Fry w/ brown rice	Burrito Potato	BBQ Lentils over greens	Mediterranean Tater	Veggie Stir Fry w/ brown rice	Pizza Potato

Chapter 5: Grocery List for One Week

To make your life easier, I have assembled the ingredient lists for each of the recipes so that you can pick and choose what you're going to make for the week and make a grocery list very easily. Adjust the quantities accordingly based on what you already have on hand, the size of your family and which options you choose (such as which version of the potato platters, etc). Remember if you decide to make substitutions such as using the link for smoothie pancakes instead of the waffles, make sure you adjust the grocery list accordingly.

Breakfast Bowl (2 servings):

1 cup rolled oats

2 Tbsp Raisins

2 Tbsp Dried apricots

2 tbsp Chopped walnuts

Non-dairy milk

Granola or other cereal with as low sugar content as you can find.

Cinnamon

Banana Nut Overnight Oats (serves 3-4):

1 cup Rolled oats

1 Ripe banana

1 cup Non-dairy milk

1 Tbsp Chia seeds or ground flax seeds (optional)

1 tsp Cinnamon

½ tsp Cardamom

2 Tbsp Chopped walnuts

Guilt-Free Homemade Waffles (makes 4):

2 Tbsp Ground flax seed

6 Tbsp Warm water

2 Ripe bananas

1/4 cup Oat milk (soy and almond work great too)

2 1/2 -3 cups Rolled oats

1 tsp Cinnamon

1/2 tsp vanilla bean powder

1 Tbsp Chia seeds and hemp seeds (optional, to increase protein content)

1 1/2 cup Fresh fruit, chopped. Raspberries, mango, strawberries, and blueberries make for a delightful treat but most fruit will work great.

Chopped Salad

Spinach

Cucumber

Bell pepper

Red onion

Grapes

Berries

Cherry tomatoes

Beans

Peas

Buddha Bowl

Brown rice

Quinoa

Zucchini

Yellow squash

Winter squash

Hummus

Beans

Avocado

Tofu (optional)

Instant Pot BBQ Lentils (makes approximately 16 servings):

2 lbs Dry brown lentils, sorted & rinsed

2 Large onions, diced

3 15-oz Cans no-salt-added diced tomatoes, drained

Fresh spinach leaves, torn into small pieces, as desired

BBQ Sauce: (can also substitute your favorite pre-made BBQ sauce if you prefer)

12 oz Tomato paste

2 tsp Onion powder

1/2 tsp Allspice, optional if desired

45

2 tsp Liquid smoke

6 oz Napa Valley Naturals Grand Reserve
Vinegar

2 oz Lemon juice

For serving:

Russet, Yukon gold, or sweet potatoes

Hamburger buns

Avocado

Veggie Stir-fry:

Brown rice

Choose 4-5 of your favorite veggies:

Asparagus

Broccoli

Zucchini

Bok choy

Red bell peppers

Onion

Mushrooms

3 Tbsp Soy sauce

2 Tbsp Lemon juice

½" Fresh ginger

1 Clove of garlic

Burrito Potatoes:

Russet, Yukon gold, or sweet potatoes

Black and/or pinto beans

Corn

Salsa or fresh pico de gallo

Sautéed fajita veggies – peppers, mushrooms, onions

Your favorite hot sauce

Veggie Lovers Pizza Potatoes:

Russet, Yukon gold, or sweet potatoes

Marinara sauce

Veggie toppings: bell peppers, red onions, mushrooms, broccoli, zucchini

Black olives

Pineapple

Mediterranean Taters:

Russet, Yukon gold, or sweet potatoes

Hummus

Kalamata olives

Chopped spinach (wilted or fresh)

Cherry tomatoes, chopped

Cucumbers, chopped

Green onions, chopped

Chapter 6:
Another Helping Please!
More resources for
follow-up

If you like what you've learned and you're eager for more, or cautiously curious about the next step, please consider some of my very favorite resources for education, recipes, and more. There's a variety here, so just start with whatever calls to you. If you're a reader, there's an abundance of books. If you are a foodie at heart, start with the cookbooks and fall in love with a healthier lifestyle that way. If you're a visual learner, check out the documentaries. If you're a Cliff's Notes kind of person, check out the YouTube clips!

Whatever you do, stay tuned for future e-books and resources on www.BeansNotBambi.com, subscribe to the blog there, follow

Christin_Bummer on Instagram and on Facebook. For ongoing info and advice, join The Nourishing Life Facebook group.

Fab Five Book List (Many include recipes!)

Unprocessed - Chef AJ

The Pillars of Health - John Pierre

The Secrets to Ultimate Weight Loss - Chef AJ

Prevent and Reverse Heart Disease - Caldwell B. Esselstyn, MD

How Not to Die - Dr. Michael Greger

Healthy Plant-based Cookbooks:

Straight Up Food - Cathy Fisher

Plant-Powered Families - Dreena Burton

Bravo! - Ramses Bravo

The Health Promoting Cookbook - Alan Goldhamer

Favorite Films:

Forks Over Knives

What the Health

Eating You Alive

Best Bets on YouTube:

"How to Lose Weight Without Losing Your Mind"
- Dr. Doug Lisle

"An Introduction to a Whole Foods, Plant-based Diet" - Dr. Anthony Lim

"The Pleasure Trap—How We Got Fat"—Parts 1 & 2 —Dr. Alan Goldhamer

"Make Yourself Heart Attack Proof"—Dr. Caldwell Esselstyn

Made in the USA
San Bernardino, CA
14 May 2019